SEX
and the
CHRISTIAN
teen

JIM AUER

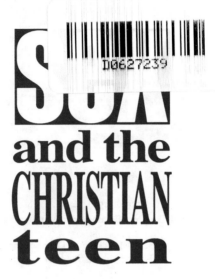

LIGUORI
PUBLICATIONS
One Liguori Drive
Liguori, MO 63057-9999
(314) 464-2500

ISBN 0-89243-632-8
Library of Congress Catalog Card Number: 94-75179

Copyright © 1994, Liguori Publications
Printed in the United States of America

Scripture quotations are taken from the *New American Bible*, Copyright ©1970, 1986, and 1991 by the Confraternity of Christian Doctrine, 3211 Fourth Street, N.E., Washington, DC 20017-1194, and are used with permission. All rights reserved.

Cover design by Chris Sharp

Table of contents

• • • • • •

Introduction: Still Another Sex Book! 5

1. Sex—Where Are We? Where Are You? 8

2. Whose Business Is *My* Sex Life? 14

3. Sex—What Are We Looking For? 20

4. A Few Pieces of You-Know-What About

   Being Sexually Active 26

5. But *How* Wrong? 32

6. Starting Over 36

7. Fallout 41

8. Sex Gone Very Wrong 47

9. Homosexuality 53

10. A Grab Bag of Good News 58

Introduction:
Still another sex book!

· · · · · ·

WELL, YOU HOLD in your hands still another Sex Book For Young People. You'll find a lot of them on the market these days. You probably couldn't live long enough to follow all the advice in all of them. Why did I write another one?

I'd like you to have a truly great sex life. That's one reason. (Sound good? I thought so.)

You're being lied to about sex in many ways. We need to stop the lies and tell the truth. That's another reason.

You deserve joy, not suffering. Sex can bring either one—no big secret about that. There are ways to increase your chances of experiencing joy, not suffering, from sex. That's another reason.

If you don't know already, you'll soon pick up the idea that this book will put God in the sexual picture.

"PUT THIS DUMB BOOK DOWN INSTANTLY!!!" a dozen voices from your memory banks may be screaming right now.

Some people have this hang-up that putting God into sex means taking all the thrills and fun out of it. They think it's like taking all the taste out of food. You end up with a sex life that's like a plate full of diet rice cakes—no sodium, no cholesterol, no fat, no calories; just healthful fiber and all the taste of fresh cardboard. They think a religious view of sex is like that.

Bull. It's a lot more like putting the real taste (back) into food. Stick around.

If any of the following descriptions fit you, You'll find something worth thinking about in this book.

- You're not sexually active, you never have been, and you don't think you should be. But you're wondering if you're normal. Or you're wondering if your lack of experience will be a handicap when the real thing, like true love and marriage, comes along.
- You've been sexually active, you still are, and so far you don't see any reason to stop. It seems like everybody does it sooner or later.
- You've never been sexually active, and you don't definitely intend to be. But it looks *awfully* interesting—especially the way some of your friends describe it—and you're wondering if it's possible to hold out.
- You've been sexually active; but now it's pretty clear that it was a mistake. You're wondering if God thinks you're scum and if you'll always be used material.
- You're sexually active with someone now, but you're beginning to have big questions about it. It isn't turning out the way you thought it would.
- You're wondering if your sexual feelings are "normal" and, if not, what kind of a life does that mean you're headed for.
- You're the victim of sexual abuse of any kind, past or present.
- You want to do the right thing sexually, but you're wondering if anybody really knows what the heck that is—or if it's even possible to find out.

"Come on, baby, light my fire."

That's a great metaphor for sex. Fire can warm and entertain and excite; it can produce marvelous, memorable good times; it can support and sustain life.

And it can burn and injure; it can run wild, cause incredible pain and suffering; it can destroy life.

Your sexuality is like that. Please consider all the possibilities, because they're there. And it's your choice. You can make it be either kind of fire. *You* can write the script for *your* sexuality.

The problem is that a lot of people are trying to hand you an already-written script for your sexuality. Why? Well, some of them just plain enjoy controlling other people. They get a cheap, superior thrill out of bragging about how they've followed the sexual script while you apparently haven't had the guts to.

Others are making big bucks off of it, selling everything from jeans to swimsuits (ever wonder why such a small amount of fabric costs so much and who's buying new Porsches with the profits?) to condoms.

So if someone, in one way or another, hands you a script that says, "You're _____ years old! You should at least have done _____ and _____ by now," inform them that you're not their robot or anybody's robot. Tell them that your body is not a performer in some teenage or young-adult sexual drama they're directing and that you'll make your own decisions.

Of course, you have to *decide* all of that inside your own mind first. You have to decide your life is worth so much that you'll write the script for it. Maybe you'll get some help to write it, but from people who honestly want you to be happy, not people who want to control your behavior or simply get into your billfold or your purse—or perhaps somewhere else.

one

Sex–where are we? Where are *you*?

· · · · ·

SEX: THERE HAVE BEEN some changes in the last few years.

Correction: Sex itself hasn't changed all that much. The human reproductive system is pretty consistent from one century to the next.

But there have been major changes in what young people hear about sex and how to handle it. Some of the changes have been great and should have happened sooner. And some have been—well, the most accurate description would be "destructive." They've caused a lot of pain.

Let's take a brief look at how the older and the younger generation communicated about sex in "the good old days" of not so long ago. Get into a pair of spiked jeans or a poodle skirt if you want to create some atmosphere, and we'll go back thirty or forty years. If we put it in sort of parable form, it might go like this:

The child was growing up and becoming more aware of the fields and plots of land that bordered on the family yard. Along one plot of land that bordered the back of the yard was a high, heavy, solid wooden fence. Adults had put up the fence. There was a gate leading to the other side, but it was triple padlocked.

"What's over there?" asked the child.

"Over where?" the adults asked in return, instantly becoming very uncomfortable.

"Over *there*, on the other side of that fence," said the child.

"Oh—uh, nothing, really." The adults cleared their throats and tried to change the subject.

"But there has to be *something*," the child insisted, "because the other day I heard that..."

"*Forget* whatever you heard! It probably wasn't very nice. There's no need to talk about what's over there for a very long time. We'll let you know when that time comes."

"Then there *is* something..."

"We'll let you know when the time comes for you to know about it. Until then, do not discuss it with anyone."

"What's the matter?" asked the child. "Is there something wrong with it?"

The adults seemed confused for a moment, but then they answered: "No, not exactly wrong, but it's—just not always—very nice. Now be a good child and just forget all about it. Even when people are grown up, if they want to be nice, they don't think about it very much."

Yes, that's an exaggeration but, in some cases, not by much. The sex topic could be delicate and explosive not too long ago.

One of the good changes in the past few decades is that many adults have become less embarrassed to discuss sex with children and teenagers. For the most part, adults no longer make up ridiculous substitute words for sexual body parts. "Penis" and "vagina" can be pronounced in public without shock waves spreading throughout a ten-mile radius.

I said many adults—not all. Some are still uncomfortable with this "new" frankness. It doesn't mean they're stupid. They just honestly think that the less something is talked about, the less of a problem it is likely to be, particularly when it comes to sex.

And there's another group of adults who are—well, almost the opposite. Your parents probably aren't among them. These people write books and magazine articles and make videos for things like high-school health or lifestyles classes. In terms of our parable, *their* approach sounds more like this:

"What's *really* over there?" asked the young teenager, pointing to a plot of land bordering the backyard. There was no fence along the border, only a sign that said, *REMEMBER. BE RESPONSIBLE!*

"Ah—you're growing up!" the adults smiled. "Tell us—are you becoming mature?"

"Of course," said the teenager.

"Well, then," said the adults, "perhaps you're ready to go over there. It's a place where people enjoy themselves in a very natural, fulfilling way. Everyone goes there sooner or later, and there's nothing wrong with going sooner—as long as you're responsible."

"What does that mean?"

"Well, there are some things you should know, so listen carefully. Along with the enjoyable, fulfilling things over there, unfortunately, there's also a cliff with a very deep drop. And some quicksand. And some poisonous animals.

"Now if you're *responsible* when you go there with someone, you won't throw that person over the cliff, see? Isn't that a good idea? Here are some other smart and responsible ideas: Try your best not to get caught in the quicksand. It could—we have to be honest with you here—change your life very drastically. And finally, try to avoid getting bitten by one of the poisonous animals."

"Are those things hard to avoid?"

"No, not really. You simply need to take some protection along with you. We'll show you how to use the protection. In fact, we'll even give you some. It's all a part of being *responsible.*"

"Does the protection always work?"

"Well, now, let's not look on the dark side. Nothing is perfect, of course, and if—well, if something happens, it's fixable. That's the part to remember. Be *responsible*, and if something happens anyway—or even if it happens because you *weren't* responsible—it's still fixable. Just come see us and we'll make it all better."

Translation: "(1) Don't rape; (2) don't make a baby; (3) don't get or spread a disease. Other than that—hey, if you're mature enough to handle it, go for it. After all, you have a right to exercise natural, healthy body functions. And if you do make a baby—no, wait, we'd better not call it a baby. Let's say if you do create a pregnancy—if you do make one of those by mistake—well, there are very simple ways of disposing of it. No problem, kids.

"As for sexually transmitted diseases, most of them are curable. Of course, some aren't, and although we don't want to worry you, *please* use your protection because we're developing kind of a big national problem along these lines…"

Not all adults are telling you that, of course. But you might easily hear it from a health or lifestyles teacher or a health textbook or video. And it's the general impression you pick up from many magazine articles and much of the media.

It's safe to say that many of your peers are going along with that message. Depending on the group you hang around with, maybe most of your friends agree with it. And the ones who are sexually active talk the loudest (along with the ones who actually aren't but want everybody to *think* they are).

Among your peers, some may flat out follow a "go-for-it" way of life. Others may insist on some standards, usually something like "As long as you *really, really* love the person and that person *really really* loves you, and you *both know it* because you can *feel it in your heart*, and you're *sure* of it, and…"

You've heard that one. You've may have heard it from people who practically hated one another six months later.

On the other side of this sex debate are probably your parents, youth ministers, religion teachers, and church leaders in general. They're saying what they've said for centuries: Wait until marriage.

Among this group, you'll find some who make a big deal about the punishment angle: Mess around sexually, even just once, and you're on a conveyor belt straight to hell, baby. That sounds terribly negative and old-fashioned, of course. But every now and then, just once in a great while maybe, you wonder if there's some truth to what they say. After all, they quote some pretty blunt Bible verses.

But it's easier and much more comfortable to dismiss these

people as narrow-minded religious freaks. After all, you've heard so often that God knows you're only human and understands and forgives and loves and etc., etc. Amen. Besides, maybe those Bible verses "were just trying to make a point for the people way back then, but things are all different now." So they don't apply anymore, right?

Other adults don't give you the sin and hell stuff, but they keep saying that sex is beautiful and wonderful and so much better if you wait and that it's really worth it to wait. Your parents probably fall in this category. They strongly and sincerely urge you to make a decision to wait—to practice abstinence (not engaging in sexual activities) until marriage.

They seem to make a good case. It does sound beautiful and wonderful to wait for the one you're in love with forever in marriage.

It may also seem next to impossible.

It may sound like someone describing the beauty and the advantages of carrying a 98.9 percent cumulative average all through high school. You nod your head and think, *Yeah. That would be nice all right, no doubt about it, and here's a big round of applause for all those rare and really unusual and sometimes really strange people who can do it. But now let's talk about my life and reality.*

And finally there are adults who still believe that it's best to wait until marriage, and they're glad they did. But they seem to have given up on that possibility for you! They sigh and say things like "I don't know—things are just different today—nothing you can do about it—but I'm afraid to think where it's all going to end up."

Big variety of opinions—*big* variety. Anything from "Go for it!" to "You'll go to hell if you do!"

So where are *you?*

Really: *Where are you* on all this sex stuff?

It's not that *I* want an answer out of you in order to judge you as an okay or a not-so-okay Christian. It's none of my business to judge you.

The point is, *YOU need an answer.*

If you say, "I'm not sure," that may work for a while, but not for very long. Situations calling for decisions about sexual behavior come early in life these days—a lot earlier and more often than they used to. You need to know where you stand *before* the windows get steamed up, *before* somebody's big brown/blue/whatever eyes turn you into the consistency of warm Jell-O.

Helping you decide where you stand is what this book is all about. And that's not easy. Sure, to some people it may seem easy. They have it all down on paper. But the chances are that they're not living in quite the same world you are. They didn't grow up in the same world you're growing up in.

It's tougher to be socially but not sexually active than it used to be. Those strange-looking guys wearing duck tails and those girls in poodle skirts you see in pictures from the fifties had the same sexual feelings you do. But they didn't have "go- ahead-do-it" messages coming at them from the soda-shop jukebox.

Right and wrong haven't changed or disappeared. But what's right has gotten more difficult to see and *still more* difficult to commit yourself to. Maybe you occasionally wonder if it's worth the hassle.

It is.

two
Whose business is
my sex life?

• • • •

WE'LL WORK AT TYING TOGETHER a couple of things in this chapter. One of them is left over from Chapter One: *Who's telling the truth when it comes to standards for sexual behavior?* We were left with a huge range of opinions—anything from "Go for it!" to "You'll go to hell if you do!"

Another is a related question. You may have heard it, and you may have felt it or even said it yourself: *What business does anybody else have telling me what to do with my sex life?*

That's a legitimate question. Let's start with that one. I think you'll agree that it makes a great deal of difference *who* the "anybody else" *is.* "Anybody else" covers a lot of ground. It even includes God.

It sounds good to say, "My sexual behavior is *my* business." And up to a point it's true. But there's a point at which it stops being true.

Let's use a different example: "My choice of a career and how I choose to make a living is my own business. After all, it's my life."

That's also true up to a point. It might be said legitimately by a young man or woman who wants to be an artist to a parent who's insisting that he or she become a stockbroker or a corporate lawyer.

But the same statement made by a bank robber is both stupid and wrong. Why? Because other people's rights are involved—and violated—in how a bank robber makes a living.

There's a point at which a person's sexual behavior involves other people, too, and that point comes pretty quickly.

So, who isn't involved—who *shouldn't* be telling you what to do?

For the most part, the people who seem to be talking about it the most—your peers and friends. Good old peer pressure. It can range from direct name-calling and deliberate put-downs about not having done it yet to a vague, indirect feeling (which you help create yourself) that you're not a fully initiated member of the group if you haven't.

If you're feeling that kind of pressure, you need to make a declaration of personal sexual independence. I know: Awfully easy for me to say, much more difficult for you to do.

But possible. Difficult, yes, but very possible. Keep your eye on the "possible"—and prepare for some pretty blunt discussion.

You don't want sex to be cheap, or you wouldn't even be reading this. But being *sexually active mainly in order to have a score story or a did-it tale to tell* is….

…well, it's about as cheap as sex gets.

In a way, patronizing a prostitute is more honest. That's payment for pleasure, pure and simple. It's awfully ugly, but there's no lying and deceitful manipulating going on.

But saying things like "I love you, you're special, you're everything to me. I need to show you how much I love you—trust me, it'll be beautiful" *mainly in order to have a story to satisfy the people who are on your case to be sexually active*—that's incredibly cheap and ugly. You don't want to do it, and you don't want to be the person who was used.

Even if you're the one who initiates the activity in order to have the story, you're being used, too—by the people who hint that you ought to do this in order to be normal and okay. (In whose opinion? Theirs, of course.)

This scene includes things that stop short of going all the way. The old "first base, second base, third base" stuff—that's sex, too. The things that precede and lead up to actual intercourse aren't exactly hide-and-go-seek. And they can be just as much using and being used as intercourse itself.

Actually, those "first base, second base, third base" terms are amazingly honest and accurate. Where do we get them? From a baseball field, of course—a *playground* where people also compete to prove their skills.

Is *that* what your body is—a *playground* for people to let off some steam, prove something about themselves, and establish a record for other people's admiration? If people are telling you to make your body into somebody's playground—or to use somebody's body as one—stop listening. You're better than that.

But does *anybody* have any business giving you guidelines for sexual behavior? Like God, for example? Let's find out.

Let's start with basic stuff, such as: There *is* such a thing as what's right and what's wrong. Another way of putting it is this: There *is* such a thing as behavior that helps people find happiness and behavior that hurts them and causes unhappiness.

If we don't agree on that much, then there's no sense going on at all. In fact, if people don't agree on at least that much, then there's no reason to form any kind of group or make any kind of agreement about anything.

Then, let's look at the evidence. Evidence—not "rules." Not what somebody said. *Evidence.* You know, *facts*—the stuff they use in courtrooms.

Not everyone will agree with this approach. "That's leaving God out of the picture," they may complain. I understand where they're coming from. But it's funny. Sometimes, leaving God out of the picture just for a few seconds can help you see very clearly *why* God is *in* the picture.

So let's go back to the first point of Chapter One. There have been many changes in what many people consider *okay* sexual behavior. Basically, what was considered wrong a few decades ago is now widely advertised as perfectly okay. After all, many people say, this is the 1990s, and intelligent people have grown out of all those stupid rules that used to tie people down and deny them their sexual freedom.

People sometimes call this the "sexual revolution," beginning with the 1960s. ("Ah tell ya, Mabel, it was them goshderned hippies what started all this mess.") Okay, if that's the right way to look at it, *then it ought to work.* Fair enough? Let's look at *the results.* If it's right, it ought to make life better and people happier.

We do that with other things, after all. For example, you really don't need any set of profound rules to tell you whether or not using drugs is a good or a bad idea. All you have to do is ask some questions. Are we better off with drugs or without them? Do they help people live a productive, happy life, or do they cause harm and destruction? Then you look at the evidence. And when you look at the evidence, you know the answer. Any idiot can see it.

You can do that in almost any area. For over half a century, quite a few governments tried to make a system called "communism" work. It was supposed to free the ordinary working people, improve their lives, and give them what was fair and just. Thousands of speeches were made and hundreds of books were written about what a wonderful revolution this was.

What *actually* happened? Repression, misery, denial of freedom—violation upon violation of basic human rights. It got so intolerable that the people themselves finally said, "This is enough," and communist governments began to fall like autumn leaves. The system collapsed. That's the *evidence,* which kind of leads you to think that it wasn't such a good idea to begin with.

Okay, let's look at all this freedom from the old rules about sex and the old way of doing things: Is it helping or hurting? *What does the evidence say here?*

Let's start with the often-heard idea that if people practice how to be sexual partners and learn whether or not they're sexually right for each other, then things will go better when they get married. We won't have people splitting up because they're not sexually compatible. That's the theory.

If that's true, then marriages in general ought to be working out *better;* the divorce rate ought to be going *down.*

But it doesn't fit the evidence. The divorce rate is going up. Some studies show that the divorce rate is higher among couples who lived together before marriage than among those who didn't!

What else do we have a lot more of? Unplanned pregnancies. Kids having babies. Teenagers forced into the role of being parents long before they're ready.

"Well, that's just tough for them. They have to pay the consequences." But we're not talking just about the teenage parents. We're talking about the babies. They have to pay the consequences, too.

I know, sometimes it seems to work out reasonably well. The seventeen-year-old mother does her best to be a good mother, and the father "takes responsibility." But nobody in his or her right mind would say this is a *good* way for a kid to start out in life.

Anything else? Abortions. That's no fun for the baby, either. Getting your body cut apart and suctioned away before you've even had a chance to live—that's the ultimate raw deal. But abortions are skyrocketing since the sexual revolution. Over a million and a half babies get cut apart and suctioned off or murdered in some other way every year. Many of them were kids of unmarried parents.

Anything else? Sexually transmitted diseases are at an epidemic level. Now, *epidemic* is a pretty heavy word—a scary word if you really understand it. The American Medical Association doesn't toss it around lightly, the way we do with words like *awesome*. When they use it, it means we've got a serious problem on our hands.

Anything else? "Date rape" and "acquaintance rape" have entered the national working vocabulary. Do you think that might have anything to do with people being told "Go for it"? Think it might have anything to with people being told they have a right to sex whenever they feel like it?

We could go on for quite a while; there are many other things. But maybe that's enough. Enough what?

Evidence.

The "new sexual freedom:" IT'S NOT WORKING. Not unless you say that sudden and drastic increases in divorce, unplanned pregnancies, abortions, sexually transmitted diseases, and rape are making life better and people happier. And we haven't even begun to mention the shattered lives that can happen without any of the above being involved.

Sure, for a few moments, there's a physical thrill. And for those wonderfully mature people who feel the need to brag about their sex lives, it gives them a story to tell. But that's not the same as happiness. It doesn't last as long, and it sure doesn't offset the price people so often pay.

"Sex—if you want it, go for it, because the old rules don't count anymore." The bottom line comes out negative. *That's the evidence.* It's also where we can bring God back in—not that God was ever away. It would be more correct to say that now we can better see why God always *was* in.

It's not a power trip on God's part. It's not God the Cranky Old Person trying to keep kids from having too much fun. It's not God the Creator who invented sex and then got embarrassed by it and tried to make it as minor a part of human life as possible.

It's God the Good Parent. When you're a parent, you won't want to see your kids hurting. So you'll probably make some rules, hoping to prevent that from happening. Your kids may not completely understand those rules at the time. Your rules may be difficult to follow at times. But you'll make them anyway. "Don't play with matches," for example, even though in themselves matches are a wonderful thing.

God is like that. That's why God has an interest in your sex life. That's why God says, "Save it for permanent, promised love; save it for marriage.

Like any good parent, God wants to see us with smiles of joy on our faces, including the incredible joy that can happen when sex goes right. God hates to see the tears and regret and emptiness on the faces of creatures for whom a gorgeous thing has turned very sour and sad and painful. So God made some rules. "This is because I hate to see you hurting."

It really is just that simple.

three
Sex–what are we looking for?

• • • • • •

NO GUY SHOWS UP at his girlfriend's house and, when her father opens the door, says, "Hi, Mr. Jones. I'm here to have sex with your daughter later on."

In spite of what many adults may think, most teen couples don't plan a date like this:

"Movie?"

"Sounds good. Pizza after the movie?"

"Sounds terrific. Sex after the pizza?"

"Why not? Fine with me."

But sex happens anyway. In fact, that's exactly what young people often say. "We didn't *plan* it. It—just happened."

In spite of this lack of plans to have sex, however, the guy frequently carries "protection" in his billfold. Which suggests that he—both he and she—at least had the possibility of sex cross their minds.

Sometimes, sex is not exactly planned but—well, pretty actively hoped for. So it happens.

But even if it was positively planned in detail ("Foreplay about ten-thirty, right after the pizza, intercourse about ten-fifty-five, on the couch in your family room, with just the lamp by the TV on?" "Sounds good."), *did they find what they were looking for?*

What *were* they looking for? Sex? Just sex? If so, they found it. No big achievement, though. It's not hidden, and the basics don't exactly require a college education.

Maybe sex *is* all some couples were looking for. That's certainly true if it was simply a case of needing a score story to tell their peers. Or if the entire experience was absolutely nothing more than an experiment in satisfying years of curiosity. But most people are looking for more than that. Far more.

You might compare sex itself to the package that was supposed to bring something. A brightly wrapped, interesting, exciting, thrilling package—but still a *package*. What people really want is something inside.

And sometimes—actually, frequently—*all they get is the package.* It's a thrill to look at it and open it up. But it's a disappointment when they realize (this may take two minutes or two years) that the package is all they ever got. There was nothing inside.

And so they're still looking for whatever they hoped to find inside. But now they have all this wrinkled ribbon and crumpled paper to get rid of and try to forget about. Sometimes yards and yards of wrinkled ribbon and huge mounds of crumpled paper.

What were they looking for? Love? That's probably at the head of the list. More accurately, they were looking for proof of love. A totally convincing, overwhelming proof that they were lovable and loved.

Having sex was supposed to be that proof. It's interesting, then, that the question most frequently asked right after sex, usually by the girl, is "Do you love me? Do you really love me?" Even when the question isn't spoken, it's often there.

Why? Sex was supposed to be proof, right? But it isn't. *Sex doesn't prove anything.* Not a thing. Including love. Does sex between a prostitute and a customer prove that they love each other?

To be blunt, the only automatic proof involved in sex is the mechanics of sex. Sex proves sex. It proves that the sex organs work. As if we didn't know that.

That may sound terribly harsh and mechanical, as though sex between human beings is not much different than sex between gerbils. I didn't say it was the whole picture. Sex can be and should be infinitely more than that.

Sex *can* be a powerful, beautiful, absolutely breathtaking *sign* of love. The key word is "can." When it is, love was there before sex; and the people involved know it.

"He/she *must* love me—we made love—that proves it."

No. Sex can celebrate. But it doesn't make and it doesn't prove.

Sometimes, what people are really looking for in the sex package is an affirmation that they're okay, that they're worth something. This is not quite the same thing as being loved, although it's closely related.

When people scratch their initials or write graffiti in all sorts of places, basically the same thing is going on. The result seems to say, "I was here. I am. I count. I can do something."

Being able to have sex, or being chosen to have sex with, seems to be proof of being okay, being worth something. But once again, sex doesn't prove that either.

Probably the most searched-for item inside the sex package is something called *intimacy*. Intimacy is a complex thing. It's being close to another person. Sharing more than just the outside of you with another person. Revealing your hopes and fears and deepest feelings. Taking risks but feeling safe at the same time. Feeling that the innermost part of you—the real you—is accepted and treasured and that you're not alone anymore.

That's intimacy. It's beautiful. And it's a very deep human need. We've been brought up to think that sex will bring that. After all, if you go "all the way," it must mean there isn't anything else of you left to share—so you must have found this wonderful, beautiful thing called intimacy. People don't think it in quite those words as their clothes are coming off; but that's the reasoning going on inside them.

And again, the package often just doesn't deliver. Why? Because people are more than their bodies—a lot more. It's really very easy to share body parts. If need be (parents will be back home in half an hour), it doesn't even take much time.

Your private body parts can be a *sign* of the deepest part of you or of someone else, but they *aren't it*. It's possible—unfortunately, very easy—to get the package (the other person's body parts) with little or nothing inside.

Two things are worth remembering about the intimacy that everybody wants with someone.

1. It takes time. A lot of time. It doesn't happen in a few days or a few weeks or even months. It's gradual, and you have to work at it. The initial "I'm in love!" rush is fun and exciting and wonderful. Nobody should put it down or call it silly. But it's not intimacy. Intimacy is later—and more difficult. Neither is finding out that you like the same kind of movies or hearing someone say, "Wow, that's rotten" when you describe the test you studied for and got a seventy-three percent on anyway. They're initial steps in the right direction, and they're wonderful. But they're still a long way from intimacy. There are no shortcuts to anyplace worth going to. That includes intimacy—and sex as an attempted shortcut.
2. You can find intimacy without sex. In fact, if you *don't* find intimacy *without* sex, it's not likely you'll ever find it *with* sex. Sex celebrates what is. It doesn't cause or create the intimacy that isn't there yet. In fact, it can even keep it from happening.

Quite a few years ago, I heard somebody say that many girls who end up pregnant really would have been happy with a good hug from somebody who truly cared and understood. When I first heard it, I wasn't entirely convinced that it could ever be that simple. So I presented the idea to a girl I had taught. Several times since she left my classroom, she had called and asked if we could talk. Two boyfriends and a baby had happened in the meantime.

She smiled and rolled her eyes a little. I can quote her words exactly because I won't forget them: "You know, if I had met somebody that really cared and if he showed it, I don't know, somehow besides the way my boyfriends said *they* wanted to show

23

they cared—I think I would have been happy just holding hands. I just needed somebody to like *me*."

Wanting to be loved, wanting to be worth something, wanting to feel intimacy—those are all good things, wonderful things, necessary things. But sex by itself, as powerful as it is, doesn't bring them or prove them.

There are still further reasons besides sex itself that motivate young people to have sex. They're not a lot of fun to discuss, but they need to be mentioned.

You may think, "It's not *that* deep and complicated. Kids just want to have fun, that's all." But this isn't purely an adult interpretation of teen behavior. Teens themselves, after a period of being sexually active, often come to the conclusion, "This is why I did it."

Rebellion or getting back at parents is one reason. Sleeping around is a vivid way of acting out resentment against parents.

If the teen thinks parents are excessively strict and restrictive, having sex is a way of saying, "Here's what I think about your stupid rules!"

Or maybe the parents have said hurting things like "You're just not the same nice kid anymore—I can't stand what you're turning into." Having sex is a way of responding, "Hey—if that's what you think about me, I may as well do it up *really* good. You haven't seen anything yet!"

Sure, the parent isn't watching and listening right at the time, and the kid doesn't announce his or her behavior. But the behavior still feels like it's making a statement. It works very well, too, if the parents find out. They're hurt, all right. But often not as badly as the teen.

Having sex is a common way of trying to keep a boyfriend or a girlfriend. No big secret here.

When you're outside a relationship, it's easy to see how weak and actually doomed this is. It's easy to realize that if it takes sex to keep a boyfriend or girlfriend interested in the relationship, then you're not worth much to that person just for yourself. It's easy to see that low self-esteem is at work here. The results pretty well speak for themselves. Putting out sex to keep a relationship going has just about the most dismal failure rate of anything around.

It's different when you're *in* a relationship and you really want it to last. It can be awfully difficult to see the same things then that you saw so clearly when you were talking about them in theory. But please keep reminding yourself of them if sex "to keep it going" starts to look like a good move.

As for people who really *are* looking *only* for sex and absolutely nothing else, they're sad. And dangerous. They see a potential boyfriend or girlfriend only through a narrow filter that calculates the possibilities for a score. Dates without sex merely lay the groundwork for dates with sex. Compliments and presents are the dues they're willing to pay in order to set up the payoff. Most of the other person's wonderful qualities aren't really appreciated—may not even be noticed.

Sex with someone like that is an incredibly empty package—no matter how exciting it feels for a while. Obviously, you deserve better.

four

A few pieces of you-know-what about being sexually active

• • • • •

LOOK AT ADVERTISEMENTS for, let's say, designer jeans, lipstick, diet cola, and sports cars. What's the message? Pretty simple: Buying/wearing/using our product will make you the center of attention from the opposite sex, bring you incredible popularity, and give you a love life that Hollywood could make into a movie.

True? Stupid question. The message is actually a myth; it's not true at all. And we generally know that. If we don't, we find out pretty quickly when the fabulous results just don't happen.

But we often buy the products anyway because—well, maybe because we're hoping that a *little* bit of the pictured results might happen after all. In other words, we buy a little bit of the myth anyway.

There are many myths about being sexually active. They're harder to see through than advertising myths. Some people believe them one hundred percent. Others sort of know better, but they're—well, hoping that some of it might be true. Or maybe nobody has ever really told them the truth instead of the myths.

There's another term for these myths. It's not as polite, but it's more colorful and equally accurate. Let's call it clumps of substance that a bull leaves lying around in the pasture. Here are a few of those pieces. The first is the biggest; it'll take a while to—step over it.

1. *Everybody's doing it.*

Everybody is almost a nothing word. Once in a while, it really does mean every human being, as in "Everybody has blood running through his or her arteries and veins."

It often means a lot less than that, as in "Everybody will be at the party!" That means the people who are important to the speaker, which might be as few as four or five people.

Every teenager is sexually active? Of course not. You know that. But how many—what's the exact percentage? Is it eighty-six percent—with the fourteen percent minority being terminally weird? Is it about seventy percent? Is it just barely over half? Is it actually only thirty-five percent or even less, and the others are just telling good stories?

WHAT'S IT TO YOU?

We'll return to the percentage question in a minute, but you need to answer the above question first. What *does* it matter to you?

It'll make all the difference in the world to you only if you're a robot who obediently takes orders from your peers.

Is *that* how you make decisions? Like *this?* "If only seventeen percent of my peers are doing something, I won't do it. If thirty percent are doing it, I'll consider it; but I may not actually do it. If fifty percent are doing it, I'll probably go along, but only if I really want to. If seventy-five percent or more are doing it, then I'll definitely do it or at least try—after all, I have my reputation to consider."

Is that how you make decisions? I hope not. You're not a piece of human silly putty that your peers can twist into what *they* think you should be. You're better than that.

Back to our original idea—the myth that every teen is sexually active. It's definitely a myth. But how many teens *are* sexually active depends on the article or the statistics you read. If you want, you can compare *People* or *Time* magazine with a sociology journal. And when they give different statistics, which do you believe?

Right here at my desk I have two articles—one stating that the vast majority of teens *are* sexually active and the other maintaining that they *aren't*. Both quote statistics and studies.

The truth is that it's different depending on the group you're a part of. You could do studies of kids in two schools in different areas of almost any large city and get different percentages. In some cases, you'd get a very high percentage and in others a rather low one.

Maybe in your school, your neighborhood, your group, your whatever, it's pretty high; so if you're not sexually active, you're one of the minority. Maybe it's the opposite—people around you may talk a lot, but most of your peers actually "haven't."

Which gets us back to the *real* question: Who the heck are *you* and what do you want *your* life to be?

If *being yourself* means something to you, the "sexually active" statistics won't mean anything at all to you. As for the actual myth—it is a myth. *Not* everybody is doing it.

2. *If you're not sexually active, you're probably gay or maybe sexless or something weird like that.*

Total stupidity in this one. I mean, this myth actually *works hard* at being stupid and brainless. The twisted "logic" behind it goes something like this: To be normal, people have to begin doing something just as soon as they're physically able. In short, if you got it, you gotta use it. Otherwise, there's something wrong with you.

You can disprove this with a zillion examples. Here's one: Walter Payton, probably the greatest running back ever, didn't get into organized football until the tenth grade. Before that, he was in the school band. Was there something *wrong* with him before tenth grade?

3. *Being sexually active makes you a better sexual partner. Since you're more experienced, you're more relaxed and confident; and, of course, you know more about what to do.*

Wait a minute! Isn't sex supposed to be about love? This sounds like a *performance*. This sounds like something that's going to be judged and rated. ("Jack averaged 9.3 for sexual artistic merit but only 8.2 for technique. Jill, however, had an outstanding night even though her partner was a little off—9.6 for artistic merit and 9.8 for technique!")

Looking at sex in this way puts it in a category with figure skating, where the performer finishes a well-practiced routine and then anxiously awaits the judges' numbers.

It's a mechanical, nerve-endings approach to sex, with love out of the picture. What do you say at the beginning of a potential session: "I'd like to practice with you so I get really good at it"? (At least that might be more honest than "Let's make love.")

Not only does this myth turn sex into mechanics, it does the exact opposite of what it says. Putting a "performance factor" into sex definitely does *not* make for a relaxed, confident outlook. It makes for a nervous, self-conscious, "I hope I'm good" approach, which any married person will tell you can positively *ruin* sex.

4. *It makes you better able to have a good sex life and a good marriage when you do get married.*

So why do people who have slept around a lot and couples who have lived together before marriage have a *higher* divorce rate?

5. *You have to have sex. You can't do without it. Once you're past or even just into puberty, it's abnormal not to have sex.*

What a slap this is at all the single people in the world who don't sleep around! Think of the millions of unmarried people in the world. This includes not just priests, Brothers, and nuns, but all widows and widowers and other people who, because of a demanding career or any other reason, have chosen to remain single.

The above myth says that every single one of them either (a) sleeps around or (b) isn't normal! Is that fair? Is that accurate? You know better.

What about the married person whose spouse is injured or seriously ill for a long time or is overseas in the service? In cases like that, we expect such a person to be faithful—which bluntly means not having sex.

Most people in that situation *are* faithful. But according to this myth, their beautiful, loyal, loving faithfulness is simply a case of being sexually abnormal. What an ugly, cheap shot. This myth is full of more garbage than New York collects in a month.

6. *Once you've had sex, you can't go back to not having it, at least not for more than a very short time.*

More garbage. *Many* people do. This includes married people in situations such as we mentioned above, *and* it includes dating couples who realize that sex should not be part of their relationship.

Sexual experience is a very strong thing, yes. Putting a stop to it is difficult, yes. But this myth treats it like an irreversible addiction. ("Once you've had sex, you're a sexaholic, and you'll always be that way—there's no cure.") It isn't.

7. *Being sexually active shows you're not a little kid anymore.*

Actually, it may easily show the opposite—that you *are* emotionally very much a little kid with a set of operating adolescent sex organs.

What are little kids like? Really little kids. They're full of one major attitude toward life: "I want." They see something attractive, and they do their best to get it. It may or may not belong to them, it may or may not be good for them, and this may or may not be the right time for it. But that doesn't matter. They don't think in those terms. When a kid is still little, "I want" automatically means "I'll go get."

That's because they're still little. It's kind of expected then. But you're supposed to grow out of it. When "Go for it!" automatically follows "Looks like fun!" this is not adult behavior. It's the kind we call juvenile or even infantile. Unfortunately, it's possible to act that way at any age.

8. *After a few dates, especially if the other person shows you a really good time, you sort of owe them at least* something *sexual.*

If you're an official prostitute and somebody puts the right amount of dollars in your hand and you put the dollars in your pocket, then, by the rules of a business deal only, you "owe" them sex. That's the only case of "owe."

Owing sex has nothing to do with a dating relationship. Yet some kids have anxiety attacks over how much they're "supposed" to put out after which date or which week in the relationship! Talk about being a slave to somebody else's degrading rules.

And who made up this myth, these "rules?" People who see others as an opportunity to score. People who see sex as a thing to be given or traded in return for something.

If it were written out or actually spoken, it would go like this: "If I go with you for a couple of months (doing you a favor), you owe me. If I spend some bucks showing you a good time, you owe me. If I'm an Ultimately Cool Person around school or if I have a fabulous body and you're sort of ordinary but I pay attention to you anyway, *you owe me.* You owe me the most personal thing you have." What would you say to someone *who actually spoke those words to you?*

Thought so.

So don't go along with someone who's saying those words to you with actions or disguising them with sweeter, more indirect words that mean the same thing.

But *how* wrong?

• • • • •

DOES GOD REALLY SAY it's wrong? How do we know? Did he really mean it, or at least wasn't that just for a long time ago? Just exactly how wrong is it—enough to send you to hell for? Seems like some people think this is THE sin, the worst one of all, but is that really true?

Let's start at the top of the list. Does God really say that sex outside of marriage is wrong? Did that idea come from God or from a bunch of dried-up old church people who were scared of sex or somehow were turned off by sex or were just born sexually weird?

You want the bottom line, right? Yes, it's awfully clear that this is God's position. And it's not that God is narrow-minded. In Chapter Two, remember, we looked at God's reasons for getting involved in people's sex lives. It's definitely not that God is antifun or doesn't understand people or just likes to boss them around.

Let's start with a passage that is about as clear as you can get: "Let marriage be honored among all and the marriage bed be kept undefiled, for God will judge the immoral and adulterers" (Hebrews 13:4).

Another passage that puts it both clearly and bluntly is "Be sure of this, that no immoral or impure or greedy person...has any inheritance in the kingdom of Christ and of God" (Ephesians 5:5).

Here are a few more. (They're often phrased in male terms, because it was the custom of the time they were written in, before the use of inclusive language became an issue. But they're meant for everyone.)

Avoid immorality. Every other sin a person commits is outside the body, but the immoral person sins against his own body. Do you not know that your body is a temple of the holy Spirit within you, whom you have from God, and that you are not your own? For you have been purchased at a price. Therefore glorify God in your body.

1 Corinthians 6:18-20

This is the will of God, your holiness: that you refrain from immorality, that each of you know how to acquire a wife for himself in holiness and honor, not in lustful passion as do the Gentiles who do not know God.

1 Thessalonians 4:3-5

Therefore, sin must not reign over your mortal bodies so that you obey their desires. And do not present the parts of your bodies to sin as weapons of wickedness....

Romans 6:12-13

Let us conduct ourselves properly as in the day, not in orgies and drunkenness, not in promiscuity and licentiousness, not in rivalry and jealousy.

Romans 13:13-14

Some people try to argue that those rules were meant just for people back then and that they have little or no application today. Actually, the sexual social climate at the time was amazingly similar to today's.

Many people regarded sex simply as a natural need, something like food. Their rule for sexual conduct was similar to the guideline many people use today: *As long as nobody gets hurt (as in rape), what's wrong with it?* Sort of like *As long as you don't rob or kill somebody for food, what's wrong with eating?*

But that's not how God views it. We could take the next couple of pages or so quoting further Bible verses, but it's probably not the best approach. People who aren't moved by four or five Bibles passages on a particular topic aren't likely to be moved by thirty or forty.

Not every case of sex outside marriage is on the same level of seriousness. *(Sex* here can mean actual intercourse or petting and fooling around so heavily that it produces the same or nearly the same reaction as intercourse.)

Take the cases of sex between rapist and victim; between two married people having an affair; between two teenagers who are deliberately doing it so they can have a score story to tell their friends; between two other teenagers who, without actually intending to, let their hormones get into an almost unstoppable rush; and, finally, between a young couple who are deeply in love and engaged to be married in a few weeks.

Each of these is a case of sex outside marriage. Are they equally serious? Obviously not. The first and last cases, for example, are hardly in the same ballpark as the others.

So there's a great range of seriousness or sinfulness. But once that becomes apparent, some people immediately want to know "Where's the point at which it becomes REALLY, REALLY bad? How bad does it have to be for God to send you to hell?"

Those questions assume that you can take every instance of sex outside marriage, including everything that was going on in the minds and emotions of the two people involved, and plug it into some sort of a computerized morality program that would then spit out the analysis: "This particular act of extramarital sex ranks 6.8 on a scale of 1-10. The cutoff point for going to hell is 6.5, so these two are definitely in trouble."

In one sense, the question is hardly worth trying to answer. It's often a disguised way of admitting, "I want to get away with as much as I can, so how much *can* I get away with before God seriously busts me? If it takes a 6.5 rating on the extramarital sex scale to go to hell for, I'll stop at 6.4 or maybe 6.3 to be sure."

That's playing cat-and-mouse games with God, which is not exactly the idea of trying to live a Christian life. It's more like a little kid who has been told not to take any cookies until after dinner, but he tries to figure how many he can probably take and eat anyway before Mom gets so mad she grounds him for a week.

Notice that the classic "How far is too far?" discussion usually centers around *actions*—and resulting *re*actions in the body of the person performing the actions, obviously.

Just actions.

Not persons.

There's the mistake in attitude right from the start. "How far can I go" usually means "How much pleasure can I get in my body from doing things with another person's body before it really makes God mad?" That turns the other person into a tool and his or her body into a plaything.

That's where the essential wrongness lies. The sexual parts of our bodies were created to say "I love you forever" to someone to whom we've promised ourselves forever and to help create new life—new human beings—that our shared love can nurture and care for.

Are sexual sins *the* sins—the bottom of the moral slime pit in the eyes of God? Well, the Bible has some pretty tough things to say about them, but it doesn't have tunnel vision. The prophets of the Old Testament probably thundered more about injustice to the poor and helpless than about sexual fooling around. The parables of Jesus focused a lot more on justice and mercy than on sex.

But that doesn't make sexual misbehavior into small stuff—certainly not when it comes to consequences. They can be pretty large—and downright permanent. But that's another topic.

six
Starting over

• • • •

YOU'RE DRIVING DOWN, let's say, Interstate 37. (Don't look for it on a map. There isn't any; this is a story.) You're on your way to a destination that has been described as absolutely marvelous. Not easy to arrive at, but marvelous. Definitely worth getting to. When you began the trip, you had every intention of staying on I-37, and for a while, everything goes exactly "the way it's supposed to be."

And then the interstate seems to get a little boring. You wonder if maybe taking a different road, kind of a scenic side road, at least for a while, might be—well, more fun. After all, you basically know what direction you're heading in. Can't be much of a risk, right?

So you do. An exit and a couple of quick turns later and you're on something called Old Barn Hill Road—and darned if it *isn't* fun! Some great sharp curves and hills and dips give you that pleasant little flutter in your stomach. And scenery—yes, yes! What scenery!

But after a while—maybe a short while, maybe a long while—Old Barn Hill Road isn't quite so much fun anymore. You have to work at following it. The curves and hills and dips don't sit so well inside your gut anymore. The scenery—well, it's still interesting enough, but you've seen it before. It's not exactly a brand-new thrill.

You also have the feeling that the road is taking you away from the direction you wanted to travel in.

On top of everything else, Old Barn Hill Road isn't paved anymore. It's gravel—rough, bumpy gravel—and big sections of it have washed out. You barely missed going over the edge into a nasty ditch a short while back. And then comes a faded wooden sign along the side of the road: "Bridge Out 10 Miles." It's starting to get pretty obvious that taking the side road was a real mistake.

So you just keep driving down Old Barn Hill Road, right? Because once you're on it, you may as well stay on it, right? And if the sign is right and you come to the bridge that's out and go over the edge onto some rocks or into a river a hundred feet below— well, that'll be a shame, but what else can you do, right? Or maybe you just stop and stay where you are because there's no going back—not anymore, right? Old Barn Hill Road is a one-way street. Or things might turn out just fine even if you keep heading down the road! That sign was probably wrong. If you keep driving, Old Barn Hill Road will probably lead you right back to the expressway, right?

OF COURSE NOT!

We're talking sex, of course, not traveling. By now, you've figured out what the road illustrates: making a mistake in sexual behavior. It's not a perfect illustration (it's not meant to put down real country roads!), but many things in the analogy fit pretty well.

Almost every sexual "side road" trip begins with some great scenery (don't have to explain that, do we?), an apparently exciting change of pace from staying straight, some enjoyable physical sensations...followed by the realization that this isn't working out so well after all. Then come moderate to massive regret and wishing it were possible to start over.

Is it?

Sure.

Is it easy?

Depends.

To continue the example, it depends on how far down the side road someone went and what happened along the way. It depends on how strongly the person wants to get back on the highway. It may depend on whether or not they're willing to talk to someone about the situation, if need be, and get help in making it back.

A mistake in sexual behavior can involve going too far but not all the way, with the resulting feeling of being slightly used, cheap material. Or it might be having gone all the way many times and having a couple of kids, perhaps by different partners, as part of the results. You can see how "the journey back" is going to be pretty different in those two cases and many others in between.

Obviously, it's better—and certainly easier—not to have to make a journey back. But in case you do—or in case anyone you know does—let's talk about starting over.

Let's start with God and with the Gospel of John, Chapter 8, the story of the woman caught in adultery. You've probably heard this story more than once. If not, or if the memory is faded, look it up—right now, if possible.

Many people wonder what it was that Jesus wrote in the sand. We'll never know, at least not in this life. It's an interesting question, but the answer isn't important. The result is that Jesus ends up facing the woman who had been literally caught in the act, led out in public, and made to stand there in front of everyone. Imagine her feelings of shame, regret, anger, and fear!

Whatever Jesus wrote made the woman's accusers decide they'd be more comfortable somewhere else. So now it's just the two of them. She doesn't know Jesus is literally the Son of God, the Messiah, but she knows Jesus is regarded as a prophet. Prophets could be awfully tough on sinners. Even with the others gone, she's an emotional basket case.

Jesus acts accordingly. No sermon, no finger pointing. Instead, he starts asking some really silly questions. "Where did they all disappear to?" As if he hadn't seen them leave! "Has no one condemned you?" Good Lord, that's exactly what the whole crowd had been doing—and probably enjoying it!

The questions are so playfully silly that she finally gives a really silly answer to the last one. "No one, sir." Right.

Jesus says, "I won't, either."

Now it's not that Jesus thinks this is small stuff. He never said that. He didn't say, "Well, it doesn't really matter." After he lets her know she's forgiven, he's definite about the action: "From now on, avoid this sin." He doesn't whitewash it, either—he says "sin" very plainly and bluntly.

But he does forgive. Instantly and with great understanding.

The gospel doesn't say what happened after that. We would like to think, of course, that the woman began "the journey back," knowing that, in God's eyes, she *was* back.

But that doesn't mean she had no worries and nothing to take care of. Chances are, there were quite a few things—like breaking off the relationship, worrying if she was pregnant, reestablishing her reputation, and finding someone (or refinding her husband, perhaps) to love her in spite of everything, which was certainly pretty public by then.

God forgives the sin—always. But God doesn't change diapers. God doesn't magically change public opinion and reestablish reputations. God doesn't instantly cure sexually transmitted diseases or cancel their consequences. God does give the strength to get through all those things.

As with any other sin or mistake, if you make it once, do you have to keep making it the rest of your life? Of course not. What if you make it ten or twenty or thirty times—*then* do you have to keep making it forever? Of course not.

If you tell a lie shortly after you learn to think and speak, are you doomed to be a professional liar for the next seventy or so years? Of course not. At any moment, you can decide to change and be whatever kind of person you want to be. The longer and more often you've acted differently can make changing more difficult, but it certainly doesn't make it impossible.

True, once physical virginity is gone, it's gone. And that's not small stuff. It would be a great mistake to look at virginity or lost virginity and say, "Oh, well—not that big a deal." It *is*. And because it is, starting over may seem futile. "You can't go *back* to being a virgin." No, but you don't have to stay sexually active—or open to the next opportunity—either.

It's kind of like this: Two people rob separate stores. One decides it was a huge mistake. He tries to make up for it, decides he's never going to do that again, and he doesn't. The other decides it was an exciting way to make some quick cash. Whenever she enters a store, she checks out the possibilities for how easy it might be to rob.

It's now a couple months later. At the moment, neither person is robbing a store. But one is looking for the next available opportunity; the other has decided he never will again.

Both people at one time robbed a store. But right now, one is still a thief; the other is an honest person. True, he can no longer say, "I've never stolen something," but he can rightly claim to be an honest person who will continue that way. That's awfully important.

It's similar with sexuality (with one huge difference: robbery is always wrong; sex is not!). This is sometimes called secondary virginity. It means deciding to reserve sex until marriage after having been sexually active one or more times. "That was then, this is now."

It has a lot to do with forgiveness. First of all, God's. You have to seek it and believe in it. That's a lot easier than the other parts.

You may need to ask forgiveness of your partner if you were principally the one who pushed being sexually active. You be the judge of whether that will help heal or not. If the very sight or sound of you sends that person into a frenzy of anger, it might be better to ask forgiveness through God.

Then you need to *do* some forgiving. You may need to forgive the other person if he or she pushed being sexually active. It may not come quickly or easily, but work toward it and ask God for help with it. Grudges, including grudges over sexual activities that were a mistake, are like baggage that weighs you down when you're trying to get on with your life.

Finally—for some people, this is the most difficult of all—you need to forgive yourself. If you need to start over and want to start over, the very fact that you want to shows what a good person you are. Believe in that.

And if at the present time you *don't* have to start over, don't do something to make it necessary.

seven

Fallout

• • • • • • •

IN 1958 A RATHER DARING (for its time) movie called *High School Confidential* featured a dramatic scene in which a teenage boy goes looking for his girlfriend and finds her in the school library searching through a medical encyclopedia. As he bends over her shoulder, he sees the book open to the entry titled *Pregnancy*. She turns to him with fright written all over her face and whispers, "They don't tell you how to stop it."

That was 1958. Today, a scene in which the teen couple at least considers abortion would probably follow shortly.

The final scene, which a teen magazine of the time called "beautiful and inspiring," shows the girl sitting alone on a bus. Remember, it's 1958; she's going *away* to have her baby so the neighborhood won't find out about it. Her boyfriend walks down the aisle of the bus with a strong, supportive smile on his face and sits next to her. They're going to face the future together. In other words, it's all going to work out.

Does it? Well, the movie ends there. More importantly, what about real life? Does it all turn out okay in real life.

This chapter is about the consequences of teen sexual activity. If you're like many of your peers, right at this moment a feeling inside you is saying, *Yes, yes, yes, you've told us this a hundred times. We know what the score is. And we know all the possible consequences of scoring, too. It's like 'Just say no.' We've heard it.*

We'll try to say it a little differently.

You might also be thinking, *Here come the scare stories.*

Yes and no. There are two kinds of scare stories. One kind is made up—invented or at least exaggerated—usually by adults to get kids to behave the way the adults want them to. The classic Boogeyman, for example. "Don't _____ (whatever) or the boogeyman will get you."

But there's a second kind of "scare" story: simply, flatly telling about scary things that really are there—not invented or slanted or exaggerated. Just plain *there* and very real. Only a seriously dim-brained adult tells the first kind as a cheap tactic to influence young people's behavior. Only a wimpy, seriously irresponsible adult does *not* tell the second kind.

"We won't get pregnant, we won't get pregnant, we won't get pregnant." But it happens a million and a half times every year to teenage couples.

"And even if we did, it would still work out because we love each other." But only a few of those million and a half unplanned pregnancies lead to lasting, love-filled marriages.

You may know of someone who is making unplanned parent-hood work out as well as possible. When that happens, everyone involved deserves a medal. It's not easy adjusting to a baby, even for a married couple who positively planned the baby! People who are doing everything to make it work out in less than those circum-stances are exceptionally good, strong people. The last thing we want to do is to make them seem second-class people or second-class Christians. And yet—*it didn't have to happen.*

Particularly sad are situations where it just isn't working out well at all. That didn't have to happen either. *An unplanned teenage pregnancy just isn't fair to anyone.* Particularly not to the baby who gets sliced apart limb by limb, suctioned out, and thrown away at an abortion clinic. About a third of all abortions in the country are performed on teenage mothers, many who were opposed to abortion—before they got pregnant.

What happened? Mix these ingredients together: A frightening, drastically life-altering situation; the prospect of career plans scrapped or put on indefinite hold; often a realization that the baby is the result of temporary passion, not permanent, committed love (also known as finding out that the father of the baby is a jerk); the financial or emotional inability (or both) to care for the baby.

Add to that the persuasive voice of someone who seems to understand and who says things like "Listen—everyone makes mistakes. We're all human. Things happen. But one mistake doesn't have to ruin your future. That's not being fair to yourself. Abortion is a simple procedure and takes only a few minutes. Isn't it time to put this behind you and get on with your life?"

Sounds pretty good, doesn't it? Especially if you're scared and upset to the point of being desperate. *That's* why girls who give antiabortion speeches can end up having an abortion.

It's not fair to the former mother, either. The possible physical complications of an abortion—anything from sterilization to death—are in tiny fine print on a piece of paper that she will probably sign without ever having read it. If they turn up in her body—well, she knew what she might be in for. That signed paper proves it, right? It's still unfair three years later when she sees three-year-old kids at a playground and starts sobbing and wondering what her kid would have been like.

It's unfair to the baby if it grows up seeing Daddy once a week or once a month—or maybe never—instead of every day. More than one kid grows up with this memory of Daddy: "I saw a picture of him once." That really hurts.

It's unfair to the father if he would like to see the baby every day, or at least often, but the relationship with the former girlfriend is now so strained and bitter—almost turned to hatred—that it just can't be worked out. That's pretty common.

It's unfair to the grandparents, who end up doing a lot of the baby raising at a time in their lives when they were finally looking forward to a little breathing space, a little time for themselves, after years of raising their own family. Now there are diapers and feedings all over again.

All through this, the baby is cute and lovable and deserves everyone's love. But that doesn't make everything right or easy.

"I won't get a disease, I won't get a disease, I won't get a disease." But a July 1992 report from the World Health Organization cited 350,000 cases of sexually transmitted diseases occurring every day. Yes, you read that right. 350,000. Every day. We could list more statistics, but they change all the time—almost always going *up*—so there's little profit in it. The point is that many sexually transmitted diseases are now being called "epidemics," and that's not a scare word doctors and scientists toss around lightly just to be dramatic. Things have to be genuinely bad, virtually out of control, before something is officially labeled an epidemic.

The scariest, of course, is AIDS because it's fatal—unless a stunning breakthrough happens shortly. Even if that does happen, it's likely that AIDS will become a "chronologically manageable" rather than a curable disease. This means that the person may not die from it, but he or she will still have it, still be sick from it.

AIDS and diseases related to HIV (the virus that causes AIDS) are now the *leading* cause of death among young men in several states and many major cities. Just a decade and a half ago, the disease was so new it didn't even have a name. No matter how you cut it, that's scary. And it's not made up.

Why the incredible "wildfire" spread? Because HIV (human immunodeficiency virus) is not like, for example, the flu virus, which acts pretty quickly. When that enters your bloodstream, it's not long before your head pounds, you're achy all over, and your digestive system is doing nasty, reverse-order things. From point of entry to point of feeling sick is a matter of hours.

HIV can enter someone's system and not show any signs of being there for years. He or she looks fine, feels fine, acts fine. Fine enough, for example, to have sex. He or she won't know anything about being HIV positive without having blood tests run and during that time can transmit HIV to any sex partner—whether homosexually or heterosexually.

Some people feel immune to AIDS because "I'm not gay." HIV doesn't say, "I can't go in this bloodstream—this person is straight!" AIDS is not an exclusively homosexual concern. In some areas of the world, the number of straight people with AIDS equals that of gay people with AIDS.

There are well over twenty other sexually transmitted diseases (STDs) besides AIDS. Some have also been declared epidemics. Some are also incurable, such as genital herpes. Some are particularly sneaky, such as chlamydia. Men may have no symptoms, yet they can transmit the disease. Most women will notice nothing until complications from the disease set in.

Some people see sexually transmitted diseases as God's punishment for forbidden sexual activity. STDs are no more a direct punishment from God than an unplanned baby is. The two cases are very different, obviously. But they're alike in that they're very possible results of sexual relations that shouldn't be taking place. God doesn't directly make those results happen. God doesn't step in and stop them, either.

There is, of course, the Great American Condom Solution! It goes something like this: "Hey, kids, gather around and let us Concerned Adults tell you how to be responsible and protect yourself when you're having fun! Listen, we know you're going to do it—you just can't control yourselves, right? But you've also probably noticed that we have a couple of nasty little problems developing in our country. Diseases going around and around, just an awful ot of babies that nobody really planned for—that kind of thing. We really ought to cut down on those things, you know.

"So let's hear it for *Safe Sex!* Or *Protected Sex!* Call it what you want, just do it—uh, we mean do it 'with protection!' Wear that condom! Or, if you'd prefer, swallow that pill (regularly, remember—don't miss a day)! Then you can just—well, you know, feel almost worry-free—and socially responsible, too!"

What a pathetic, pathetic, pathetic joke.

In the past couple of decades, millions upon millions of dollars have been poured into "safe sex" education programs and materials of all kinds. Why? To cut down on teenage pregnancies and sexually transmitted diseases. What has happened to both since then?

They've gone *up* almost off the scale. Talk about a massive, monumental failure. "Safe sex for teens" almost wins the award of the century in that category. The only bigger failure I can think of at the moment is Communism's promise to make things better for the ordinary working person. As Molly Kelly, a dynamic and popular speaker on chastity for young people, puts it, "safe sex" programs only give young people the tools (therefore the approval and encouragement) to do the very thing that's causing the problems.

Completely safe sex? No such thing. Even the safe sex people admit that. They have to. There's a mountain of statistics proving otherwise. The only safe sex is waiting for the person who has also waited for you. Then it's a lot more than just safe.

There's another huge flaw in the "safe sex" viewpoint. It goes like this: No baby + no disease = no harm. That reduces you to a set of operating reproductive organs. If nothing goes wrong down there, what's the problem?

So if you find out you've given your virginity to someone you now realize is a jerk, there's no harm done. After all, it was "safe sex!" (No baby, no disease—remember?)

If you find out that your body was mostly material for curiosity or a score story to tell peers, there's no harm done. After all, one or both of you used responsible protection!

In other words, when it comes to safety, your feelings, your self-esteem, and your soul don't count.

If I sound angry here, it's because I am. I've held too many sobbing young people on my shoulder who had listened to the "safe sex" and "go ahead—everybody does" lies.

Lies.

God has a better idea for sex. We really need to listen to it. And it's possible. It really is. If it weren't, God wouldn't have given it to us.

eight

Sex gone very wrong

• • • • • •

IN THE SUMMER OF 1993 the massively flooding Mississippi, Missouri, and other rivers turned life into a nightmare for hundreds of thousands of people. The very waterways that once built the economy of the area went out of control and wrecked it. Anything so immensely powerful is capable of great accomplishment and great destruction: water, wind, fire. And sex.

This chapter has unpleasant topics. "Lilies that fester smell far worse than weeds," Shakespeare wrote. Something originally very beautiful, which then somehow goes wrong, ends up far uglier than something that wasn't pretty to begin with. That's a good description of the results when sex turns into sexual abuse, incest, rape, and pornography.

At this moment, our readers have separated into two divisions: those to whom something has happened and those who are only reading about it. There's something in this chapter for both, including guys.

If you've never been a victim of any kind of sexual mistreatment (which includes many things besides actual rape), it's almost certain that you know someone who has—even though you may not be aware of it. Statistics in this area keep changing, nearly always for the worse; but it's currently estimated that one in every three or four girls and one in every six or seven boys will have been abused at least once by age eighteen.

Some adults, nearly always male, see children and adolescents as sex objects. It's not clear how or why the beautiful desire to be lovingly, sexually united with someone gets so twisted (which is exactly what the word *perverted* means in Latin); but it happens, apparently more frequently than we would care to think about.

When the adult acts out these urges, the result could involve full intercourse or touching and fondling of sexual parts. Notice we didn't say "*simply* touching." There's nothing simple or small about being sexually used in any manner.

If the child is rather young, he or she may not realize the actual sexual dimension of the actions. The adult may even convince the child that these things are actually legit but not something we talk about later. A young child may even find it enjoyable and somewhat exciting.

With an older child, when the actions may include full intercourse, the offender may also try to convince the victim that this is actually very normal activity. It's just that people don't talk about it. This often happens in the case of incest, which is sexual abuse, usually including intercourse, by a person in the victim's family.

Seldom is the offender a stranger. The pervert who jumps out from behind the park bushes and grabs a child is responsible for only a tiny percentage of sexual abuse of children. The offender is nearly always someone well known to the victim. It's often someone the victim admires, likes, even loves—and sometimes depends on. That's why it can happen so often.

If it's happened to you sometime in the past...

First of all, it was not your fault, no matter how ashamed or angry or stupid you may feel now. If you were very young and didn't realize the sexual dimensions of what was going on at the time, you might feel that you should have. Now that you do realize that you were being sexually victimized, you're furious at the offender and angry at yourself for not being smarter.

You might also feel extremely ashamed and stupid if, at the time, it felt good and you sort of enjoyed it. That means your body was working the way God made it. Any kind of sexual touching, unless it's violent, is going to feel good.

The responsibility is totally on the adult. Always. A social worker once told me, "I don't care if a child parades in front of an adult naked. Every adult knows that sex with a child is wrong and can decide not to do it."

Once again, for the record—and please believe it one hundred percent—no matter what the circumstances, *it was not your fault.*

Second, you have some baggage to deal with—but you have *not* been ruined. That's actually a two-part statement. Let's start with the second part.

There's a difference between having a scar, a bad memory, and being ruined. You're still the same wonderful person you've always been. You're not dirty, you're not bad, you're not used material, you're not sexually second or third rate. You can have a wonderful, loving sex life with the spouse who will choose you to spend his or her life with. If you're a boy who was abused by a man, you have not been made homosexual or infected with sort of a psychological virus that will make you homosexual at some future time.

But you do have some baggage to deal with and get rid of. "It doesn't bother me—not anymore" is almost always a defense against the pain that's still there. And it almost never works. Not for good. It may work for a while. Some victims of sexual abuse become so skilled at tuning out the hurt that they "repress," or *actually, temporarily forget,* the painful incident(s). This is especially true if the abuse was violent rape.

It's similar to the way the skin builds a bubble, called a blister, over a painful area. The blister protects the wounded area from further harm and enables the person to tune out the hurt while the wounded skin heals underneath.

And that's what happens—with a blister. The emotional bubble a person builds over a past incident of sexual abuse does temporarily cover the immediate pain, but emotional healing is *not* automatically taking place underneath the bubble.

Extreme anger, resentment, shame, guilt (even though not deserved), the feeling of betrayal by a trusted person, which can make it very difficult from then on to trust anyone—all those things are still there, maybe even building up.

Begin somewhere to deal with it. Talk with someone. That takes great courage because it means going back to the bubble and opening it up, which for a while will be painful. But it's necessary for healing to happen. You might begin with a school counselor, a teacher, a relative whom you know you can trust.

The first person you talk with may not be trained to help you through the process of getting rid of the hurt and baggage from the past. That can take some professional guidance. But it's a start, and that person may lead you to the professional who will help even more.

Little more than a decade ago, "date rape" or "acquaintance rape" were brand-new terms. Now they're part of the national working vocabulary. Some people are practically accustomed to it and casual about it—the way they've become about sex in general. "Date rape—yeah. There's a lot of that going on these days." It's all part of "the new sexual freedom" which some idiots maintain has made things *better*.

But date rape is not a casual thing if it has happened or almost happened to you, or if you're very afraid there's a good chance that it will.

Unfortunately, girls should make some preparations for the possibility—and I do realize how terribly grim that sounds. It may prompt a reaction like "What kind of animal do you think I'd go out with?" Problem is, no victim of date rape thought she was going out with an animal when she agreed to go out. It happened or almost happened anyway.

Resisting date rape begins with knowing that you have some weapons at your disposal. One is noise and commotion. If it's at all possible for someone to hear you, scream and don't stop. If you can break away, throw something—throw as many things as possible—

through a window. True, a public commotion around the situation will be embarrassing. But it's a lot better than being raped.

Have a law enforcement officer talk at your school to make further suggestions which play into the specific laws and regulations of your community and your state.

Perhaps best of all, take a course specifically designed for women's self-defense. Unless the guy himself is a martial arts expert, you can learn techniques to seriously discourage a potential rapist, especially one who didn't begin the evening intending to be one.

If at this point the male readers are feeling a little like, *What do you think we are?* I'm sorry. This isn't meant personally. It's just that some males really are jerks—or can be at times.

You've probably never heard of a girl physically forcing herself on a guy, but you've heard of the other way around many times. It happens. That doesn't mean it *has* to—ever. "Guys are guys, after all" is a totally bankrupt argument. Nothing *ever* justifies pressuring someone into sex, either physically or emotionally or verbally.

Dating someone who likes pornography or staying at parties where pornography is being watched—that's *really* like playing hopscotch by the edge of a cliff. Pornography portrays women as toys, things, usable body parts, not as people. In pornography, sex is rubbing nerve endings, nothing more—gerbil-level sexuality.

Few people will admit to being influenced by pornography. People who use pornography develop defensive lines just as alcoholics do. ("I can stop anytime I want.") Porn users say, "They don't really *do* anything for me; I just think they're *funny*. I like to watch how stupid it looks!"

Sure. Just like your uncle is Santa Claus.

"If you've seen one, you've seen 'em all" is another line. It's designed to make the point, "I'm not really into this stuff; in fact, it almost bores me." So why do these people keep buying or renting and watching new material?

Pornography promotes a dangerous thing called the rape myth—

that women secretly enjoy being forced into sex, no matter what they say. When they initially say "no," they don't mean it. The rape myth is a standard "plot" in one porn film after another. The story line goes from "No, no!" to "Yes, yes!" to "More, more!"

Pornography tends to make almost anything, even ugly perversions, seem exciting, enjoyable, and half normal—almost legit. Viewers are given the idea that lots of people do these things behind closed doors—and have a great time. What's the most likely conclusion from that?

This hasn't been a pleasant chapter, but today's sexual climate makes it necessary. There is one bright lining in the dark cloud of misuse and perversion of sex. God created sex in spite of the massive amount of garbage that comes from sex gone wrong. Something had to be worth that risk, and that something is this: sex is stunningly beautiful and wonderful when it goes right.

Homosexuality

· · · · ·

A YOUNG MAN I TAUGHT several years ago will never do something most guys look forward to: fall in love with a girl, get married in a lovely wedding with proud and happy parents and good friends sharing the joy, be a husband, and raise a family. No kid will ever call him "Daddy" and ask to be taken to the park or be taught how to do something or put something together—which, I can tell you, is a beautiful, wonderful feeling.

But this young man simply won't live long enough to experience that unless medical science achieves a stunning breakthrough in the very near future. Obviously, he didn't choose this, and it hurts.

Another young man I taught several years ago will never do any of those things either. Not because he won't live that long. Because he's gay. He didn't choose that, either; and he also has hurts from it.

That's the first point that needs clearing up about homosexuality. It's discovered, not chosen. People don't shop around for a sex to be attracted to, consider various aspects of each one, and then choose one over the other the way you might choose a Mustang over a Camaro or vice versa.

Some people may find this surprising and mind-opening ("You mean those people actually don't decide to be weird?"). Others may find it depressing ("You mean it can't be changed—even if the person wants to?").

Many theories of what causes homosexuality have floated around for years. Some have been disproved; others go in and out of favor.

Much recent research has concentrated on the idea of a *genetic,* inherited cause. It currently seems the likeliest explanation of many—perhaps even most, but not all—cases of homosexual orientation. Certainly no one can possibly choose what gets passed along to him or her through DNA.

Most straight people are rightly revolted by some of the antics that take place in "Gay/Lesbian Pride" parades in heavily homosexual cities. But those antics are not the usual reaction of someone who discovers that he or she is homosexual. The initial reaction is a universe away from "Wow, that's great! Boy, am I proud!"

Instead, the knowledge is marked by fear, sometimes almost panic, of being discovered. The person will work hard at keeping it a secret, perhaps force extra-loud laughter at gay or lesbian jokes, even though they're about as funny to him or her as an invitation to play baseball would be to a kid whose arms are paralyzed.

Often there's shame and self-doubt, too, even self-hatred. After all, the feelings that seem normal and unchangeable, as well as strong, deep, and personal, are precisely what others call sick, disgusting, and evil. That can cause some awfully heavy damage to self-esteem.

Anger comes easily, also. "Why me? What did I do to deserve this?" It's much like the anger anyone feels who has a distinct difference that keeps him or her from fitting in and doing the things others do. Anger increases when genuine efforts to change and sincere, sometimes almost desperate, prayers ("Dear God, please change me!") don't bring any results.

You don't have to approve of homosexual behavior in order to have some sympathy and compassion for a person with a homosexual orientation. In fact, sympathy and compassion are precisely what are called for by a Christian attitude. Demonstrators who carry "God hates fags" signs have a lot to learn about God. For starters, they could skim the Bible for references to homosexual behavior (less than ten), then skim it again for references to justice and charity. They'll need a calculator for the second task.

Other myths surround the issue of homosexuality. One is that all homosexuals are sex-crazed people who are attracted to practically everyone of the same sex, who exercise little or no control over their sexual urges, and who, if given the chance, would have sex with almost anyone of the same sex.

Homosexuals are not attracted to everyone of the same sex any more than straight people have sexual urges toward everyone of the opposite sex. As for having no control and hopping from one partner to another whenever the opportunity comes—yes, some gay and lesbian people do that. Some straight people do that, too.

Seeing other people simply as sets of body parts on which to exercise your sexual nerve endings—that's a sign of being a moral jerk, all right. But you can act that way if you're gay or lesbian, and you can act that way if you're straight. It has to do with your standards and your outlook on life and people, not your sexual orientation.

A final myth is that a person's homosexuality is like a disease or moral cancer that will affect—or infect—all other areas of the person's life. According to this myth, homosexuals can be expected to act dishonorably or irresponsibly sooner or later in almost every area. The facts are that homosexuals have served well in many roles, from soldiers to senators to professional football players.

That's important to remember if you should discover—or be told or entrusted with the knowledge—that someone you know is gay or lesbian. You'll be shocked at first, because he or she has probably done an excellent job of covering.

You don't have to like that particular aspect of the person. But all the rest of him or her, all the things you liked or admired—they're still there. They're still true and valid and real. They haven't been canceled or ruined or made meaningless. If in the past that person has been kind, loyal, and understanding, as well as an excellent running back or volleyball captain, he or she still is.

None of this is intended to say that homosexual activity is just perfectly fine after all. It's not intended to say that if you have strong feelings—hey, go with them and let them flow. As a moral principle, that's incredibly dangerous and wrong. In that case, people with strong interest and urges toward a career as a serial killer should feel free to follow them.

The Church's position on homosexuality is clear. Being homosexual and having homosexual feelings, attractions, and urges is not sinful. That simply follows the general principle that only *actions* can be right or wrong; feelings themselves just are. No one is morally responsible for something he or she did not cause, did not choose, and cannot change.

At the same time, the Church maintains that acting on those feelings—engaging in homosexual actions—is wrong. This teaching is based on several Scripture references as well as on the natural law, interpreted in the light of the gospels.

Natural law, simplified a great deal, basically says this: You can look at male and female bodies, study the function of the sexual parts, and conclude that God designed them to fit together—not two male or two female bodies with each other.

Most straight people have no problem with this, because it has nothing to do with their lives. "Don't have homosexual sex" affects them about as much as a traffic law passed by a city five thousand miles away. Some may even feel superior and vindictive: "Serves those people right for being strange. They don't deserve to have any fun if they're going to be like that." That's a really cheap attitude.

Some (not all) gay and lesbian people say this is not fair, that it's fine to be celibate (not have any sexual relations) if you want and choose, but that it's not fair to be *told* you have to follow that way of life. What if, some say, we're not talking about cheap one-night or one-month stands but a permanent, committed, loving relationship?

Well, they're certainly right about it not being fair. No one should have any argument with that.

On the other hand, this isn't the only case of life not being fair. It's not fair to be born with *any* condition that makes you different from most people and puts some of their activities off limits for you. It's not fair to be born blind, for example, and never see a sunset or the faces of people you love.

Every night, millions of people go to bed without decent food, shelter, and clothing—and without any chance of having them. Millions of people go to bed without safety and security, without stability in their lives, and without hope for their future. That's a lot worse and more unfair than having to go to bed without sex.

Homosexuals are not the only people expected to live a celibate life. So are all straight people who remain single. So are widows and widowers. So is the husband or wife whose spouse is too sick or injured for a long period of time, perhaps even permanently, to engage in sex.

Some young people worry that they may be homosexual for reasons that just don't add up to it. Here are some.

You are *not* homosexual simply because you haven't dated much—or at all—or if you feel clumsy and awkward around the opposite sex. Many people feel that way. And many don't begin an active, dating social life until years after others.

You're not homosexual if you have strong feelings of friendship for someone of the same sex. This is a sign of being emotionally healthy.

Guys with quiet, gentle, sensitive personalities are not gay for that reason. Girls who like rough, demanding physical activities are not lesbian for that reason, either. And finally, no one is homosexual simply because of one or even more than one experimental activity with a person of the same sex sometime back in childhood.

It's a complicated issue. We don't have it all figured out yet. What has to stop, though, is the hatred and self-hated, the ridicule and bashing. None of those things go with following Jesus.

A grab bag of good news

. . . .

WE'VE ALMOST COME to the end of Still Another Sex Book. We began with the question "Where are *you* on sex?" Actually, we're still there. The person who most needs to know the answer to that question is you. Here's an assortment of items to help you think about it.

The Good News About Who's in Charge

Being in charge of your life doesn't mean you're allowed to do whatever you feel like, either sexually or otherwise (such as knocking off convenience stores as a part-time occupation).

It means you *can* make good things happen if you want to. You *are* in charge of your life—and responsible for it. That's easy to say, not always so easy to put into practice. But it gets a *lot* easier if you truly, deeply believe it to the point where you feel it through your bones and blood and heart and soul.

You are in charge of your life. Not your friends. Not the person you're going with. Not songwriters or performers. Not movie and video producers. Not magazine publishers. Not a generic "everybody" script that some peers expect you to follow like a little robot.

You.

What do *you want* for yourself, for your life, including your sex life? What kind of foundation do *you want* to build for the family you dream of having someday? What kind of bride or groom or husband or wife do *you want* to be? What kind of role model do *you want* to be for the kids who will call you Mommy or Daddy?

What kind of preparation, what kind of dating relationships between now and then will help make that happen?

Be optimistic about these dreams! You have it in other areas. Young people will say, "I want to be a _____" and then add professional basketball player, model, business executive, heart surgeon—whatever the dream is. "It'll be tough, but I'm going to *make* it happen. I know I can do it."

Optimism and determination. Wonderful things. They *can* make dreams come true. But ask some of the same people if they plan to keep their sexuality for marriage, and you hear, "Well, I'd like to. I mean, it would be neat that way, but I don't know if it's possible the way things are these days. You know—things happen."

Career: optimism and determination—yes! Control of sex life: well, gosh, it would be nice, but…

Why this I'm-in-charge outlook on career but dunno-if-I-can outlook on sex? Here's why: Because a lot of people, including a lot of dim-brained adults have given that message. And they're wrong. Just plain flat out wrong.

Sometimes the same adult says, "If you believe it and dream it, you can do it!" about your career—and then, "Here's a condom because I *know* you can't control your sexual urges."

Tell them you're tired of being insulted like that. You're a teenage human being, not an adolescent gerbil.

And yes, once again, *you are* in charge. That includes being in charge of your own hormones.

Easy? Absolutely not. Most things worth doing (or not doing) are difficult.

Possible? Absolutely. It depends on how much you want it. It depends on how much you want to direct your own life and your own future.

What do you want your sexuality to say?

Sex is communication. It always says something, even though words themselves may not be used—in fact, usually aren't. It may say something ugly; it may say something beautiful. But it always says *something*. Here are some of the messages that sex can give. What do you want *your* sexual giving to say?

- I don't want to feel like a child anymore. Having sex with you—or at least with someone—will prove that I'm not just a little kid who doesn't know the score.
- I'm angry and I feel like breaking some rules. Your body is a very attractive place to break some rules.
- Sex is no big thing; it just feels good. Let's do each other a favor and make ourselves feel good.
- I really love you. I hope we last. If we have sex, maybe we will. Maybe sex will make it happen.
- Life is cruddy sometimes. Sex helps me forget my problems. I hope it does the same for you.
- I don't have much sexual experience, and my friends are on my case. If I make it with you, that'll be a pretty good story. They'll be impressed. I'll finally have something to brag about. My friends will think I'm normal, and so will I.
- I'm not really sure I'm likable or lovable or even attractive sometimes. If you knew all about me, you might not stay with me. But if we have sex, maybe you will.
- I love you and only you. I want to be one with you and only you forever. We've said that and promised that before God, our families, and our friends. Now let's celebrate it—again and again.

Chastity: A Step Into Freedom!

Saying no to sex before marriage is often portrayed as a restriction, a limitation of freedom. Consider that it might be exactly the opposite. Consider the freedoms that come with *chastity*.

1. Freedom from guilt and loss of self-esteem. Even people who try their best to tune out right and wrong have a lingering feeling that casual sex is wrong and that they're not quite as good a person as they were before. "Most of my friends feel guilty after they have sex, but they keep right on doing it. I don't think they're having much fun," a seventeen-year-old girl said in a *People* magazine report on teen sex.

2. Freedom from loss of virginity—the gift you could give your spouse. "I believe the greatest gift you can give your spouse on your wedding night is for that person to be your first," a sixteen-year-old boy wrote in a list of "Things I Believe"—for his girlfriend. (Yes, guys, it's possible to say that to your girlfriend. This particular guy, by the way, is also Mr. Popularity at his high school.)

3. Freedom from wondering and worrying if the person really loves you or is simply (or semi-) using you.

4. Freedom from *much* heavier bad feelings if you break up, which is never easy or fun, and which—let's be realistic—is likely, no matter how close you feel for a few teenage months or even a couple of teenage years.

5. Freedom from wondering what to say if the next person you're going with asks whether or not you've slept with someone— especially if the next person turns out to be someone you *really* hope will be a lasting relationship. "I guess if I was really serious about a girl who was a virgin—I guess I'd really wish I was too," an eighteen-year-old boy told me.

6. Freedom from deciding whether or not or how often to repeat having sex. "We did a couple times or so, but then it started coming between us," a seventeen-year-old boy told me. "It was like a pressure. When we decided to stop—period—we actually started having more fun."

7. Freedom from getting a reputation as being easy or a user. Once you have that rep, there's no problem getting partners, but there may be a problem getting someone who likes you for you.

8. Freedom from pressure to perform ("Was I good?") especially in a short time (somebody will be back home in an hour or so) and from comparing ("Was I as good as the others?").

9. Freedom from sexually transmitted diseases and everything that goes with that, like wondering if you might have one without knowing it and wondering if you should get a medical check and wondering how to arrange that (and pay for it) without anyone knowing.

10. Freedom from everything connected with contraception:
   - what kind to use
   - whether we have some with us
   - whether it worked (waiting for the next period to know if you dodged the bullet)
   - worrying about medical side effects of some types.

11. Freedom from unplanned pregnancy and everything that goes with that:
   - reaction of family and friends
   - reaction of the partner who helped make the baby
   - the abortion versus the carrying-the-baby decision
   - the adoption versus the keeping-the-baby decision

12. If keeping the baby, freedom from worry about
   - who will—really—raise the baby?
   - who's going to pay all the baby bills and how?
   - if the mother and/or father should drop or change career plans?
   - trying to have a normal teenage (supposed to be fun!) life while still being a parent
   - marriage and whether having the baby is enough basis for a working, lasting marriage
   - arranging often awkward "visiting rights" for the noncustodial parent if marriage isn't going to happen
   - looking for someone to marry who will accept the baby and be a real mother or father, even though the baby isn't hers or his

- never having to worry about the child telling that person, "But you're not my *real* Mom/Dad."

THAT IS A LOT OF FREEDOM! That's the good news about chastity. Worth going for? Worth making sure it's yours?

Your decision. Remember, you *are* in charge.

Do you have to give anything up to get it? Sure—the temporary physical thrill of sex and possibly a relationship with someone who wants sex more than he or she wants you.

Still worth going for? Your decision.

Some Nuggets of Good News From the Bible About Sex

In spite of repeatedly saying otherwise, God has gotten a bad antisex rap. God doesn't like the wrong things we do with sex (along with the wrong things we do with arms, tongues,and so forth). But God thinks sex is terrific, and that includes the rush you get from looking at someone you like and—well, appreciating. What you do later may or may not be wonderful depending on the situation, but physical attraction itself has God's blessing.

For proof, look up chapters 4 to 7 of the Song of Songs in the Old Testament. The background of this set of love poems is that a guy and a girl have fallen deeply in love and are promised to each other. At this point, don't worry about getting to the bottom of the fine points of each verse's meaning. And don't get sidetracked by the fact that the images for various body parts come from a different time and culture. Appreciation for physical beauty still comes across very clearly—with God's blessing.

Many Bible scholars believe the Song of Songs is intended to be symbolic of the love and caring that God has for the Church, for his people. That doesn't take away the blessing on sexuality; it makes it even better. When God chooses something to symbolize his intense desire to be united with us, do you think he'd choose something second rate, something really not so nice? Hardly. He would—and did—choose something terrific, something wonderful.

And look up Isaiah 62:5. Please—look it up. It's worth the few minutes it may take to find it. Once again, God uses clear, upfront sexuality as an analogy of his love for us, his passion to make us his own.

You can draw a couple of conclusions from that verse: (1) Sex as God planned it is incredibly good; (2) if God is as intensely involved with us as the second half of Isaiah 62:5 says—wow! Talk about being appreciated and desired!

Let's not throw it away by trashing the very thing, our sexuality, that God created and uses as an analogy of how he feels about us.